Make the most of each day with your loved one while you still have time. Learn to live in the moment.

ALZHEIMER'S

Where Do We Go From Here?

Lisa W. Smith

ALZHEIMER'S
WHERE DO WE GO FROM HERE?

ISBN: 1-60037-062-5 (Hardcover)
ISBN: 1-60037-010-1 (Paperback)
ISBN: 0-9768491-2-7 (eBook)

Published by:

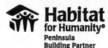

MORGAN · JAMES
THE ENTREPRENEURIAL PUBLISHER™
www.morganjamespublishing.com

Morgan James Publishing, LLC
1225 Franklin Ave Ste 325
Garden City, NY 11530-1693
Toll Free 800-485-4943
www.MorganJamesPublishing.com

**Habitat
for Humanity®**
Peninsula
Building Partner

General Editor:
Heather Campbell

Cover & Interior Design by:
3 Dog Design
www.3dogdesign.net
chris@3dogdesign.net

To my wonderful husband who believed in me when I didn't believe in myself.

ALZHEIMER'S: Where Do We Go From Here?

TESTIMONIALS

"I loved your book and read it straight through. We have walked the same journey and your book will help so many to feel they are not "walking theirs" alone. Your aunt is blessed to have you."

– Sharon

"An accurate account of the effects of Alzheimer's on the patient and their family. This book would be a definite benefit to any family just starting the journey. My grandmother passed away with Alzheimer's, and a lot of the information in this book you don't think about until it's too late, and you have missed a great opportunity to lift the burden and enjoy what few moments you can with your family member. It also makes you realize that it is okay to laugh and enjoy life."

– Jolie

"As the daughter of two victims of Alzheimer's, my sincere thanks go to Lisa for giving voice to the physical, spiritual, and emotional upheaval this disease brings to its victims and their families. We can still find moments of joy and laughter if we just look for them."

– Judy

ALZHEIMER'S: Where Do We Go From Here?

PREFACE

Alzheimer's : Where Do We Go From Here? is the story of one family's struggles with the disease. This story is written from a layman's point of view and covers various topics on the emotional, physical, and financial aspects of caring for someone with Alzheimer's. These are things learned through personal experiences about the disease's effects on persons suffering with Alzheimer's and the impact on those who love them. Trained professionals are knowledgeable of the scientific facts, statistics, causes, etc. They possess a head knowledge of the disease. Those of us who love someone victimized by Alzheimer's have a heart knowledge. We know how Alzheimer's feels. We have learned that there is sometimes a vast difference between the two perspectives. Even though trained professionals might be compassionate to those affected by Alzheimer's, we believe it is still impossible to fully understand the emotions unless one has experienced them personally. We are sharing this story and the lessons learned in hopes of helping other families who are faced with the painful realities of living with this disease. All the events in this story are real. The names of all involved have been changed to protect their privacy. While Alzheimer's is a cruel and greatly-feared disease, it does not have to rob its victims of love and respect. *Alzheimer's : Where Do We Go From Here?* will help you discover ways to add quality and dignity to your loved one's life while helping you cope with the struggles and demands placed on your family.

ALZHEIMER'S: Where Do We Go From Here?

TABLE OF CONTENTS

ALZHEIMER'S: Where Do We Go From Here?

ALZHEIMER'S
Where Do We Go From Here?

ALZHEIMER'S: Where Do We Go From Here?

CHAPTER 1

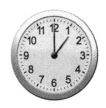

The Cold Hard Truth

ALZHEIMER'S: Where Do We Go From Here?

CHAPTER 1

The Cold Hard Truth

Alzheimer's Disease – two words capable of producing terror to the very depths of a person's soul. The fear of acquiring this disease tends to increase with age. For some of us who have a family history, fear strikes every time we can't find our car keys or forget an appointment. For us, age is not as big a factor as family history. We question ourselves frequently as we worry that we might be showing some of the early signs of the disease. A diagnosis of Alzheimer's is devastating to the victim who is coherent enough to understand what is happening and to everyone who loves him.

Alzheimer's is a condition that slowly, but ruthlessly destroys. It is a disease that robs one of cognitive abilities and memories. Short-term memory is the first casualty and then long-term memory eventually fades. It takes away the ability to perform simple, daily tasks such as dressing or feeding one's self. It gradually destroys the ability to communicate. Quality of life is greatly diminished and one's dignity is compromised. An intelligent, well-functioning person is suddenly seen as "crazy" so even his reputation suffers. With some Alzheimer's patients, a drastic personality change occurs. A person who has always been the "life of the party" may suddenly become reclusive. The grandfather that everybody loves may turn into an abusive, foul-mouthed person who frightens the grandchildren. All these changes make it difficult for friends and family to know how to react. This can lead to isolation and loneliness for the one suffering from Alzheimer's. Relationships change along with the roles played by those close to the patient. With time, incontinence becomes a problem. Sleeplessness and an unawareness of time are common symptoms, too. Suspicion, fear, anger, and sadness are among the common emotions. The costs of medical care and special living arrangements are astronomical and can create serious financial burdens for the spouse and/or family. Eventually, Alzheimer's disease leads to death.

Alzheimer's patients are not the only victims of the disease. Those who love them are also victims. It is excruciating to watch the progression of this disease on someone you love. Sadness and fear often accompany the feeling of being overwhelmed. At times, an Alzheimer's patient can become abusive and accusatory. As a family member, it hurts to be called all sorts of horrible names, be cursed at, or accused of wrongdoing. Even though you know it's the disease talking and not the one you love, it still hurts. If the present is this difficult, you worry how you will handle the future as the disease brings further deterioration. If this now runs in your family, does that mean your chances of developing Alzheimer's are greater, too? That thought creates its own terror. How will you ever deal with all that will be required of you? Can you handle the bills and financial decisions as well as all the medical decisions? Will it all be too overwhelming? How will you balance your new responsibilities with your old ones? Will everything in your life change? How will you survive as your loved one slowly slips away from you? Depression can be a common side effect for the family members, and particularly, the primary caregiver. A diagnosis of Alzheimer's can change more lives than just the one with the disease. It seems that in some ways, it is the family who suffers the most.

Alzheimer's is a disease that is affecting millions in the United States. According to the Alzheimer's Association, the number of people living in the U. S. who have Alzheimer's has reached 4.5 million. This has more than doubled since 1980. This number is expected to grow until it ranges between 11.3 million and 16 million in 2050. A Gallup poll commissioned by the Alzheimer's Association found that 1 in 10 Americans said they had a family member with the disease and 1 in 3 knew someone with Alzheimer's. The risk of developing the disease increases with age. One in 10 individuals over 65 is diagnosed and nearly half of all individuals over 85 are affected. In some rare cases, people in their 30's and

40's have been diagnosed.[1] Alzheimer's is a far-reaching disease that will continue to touch families.

Our family is currently on the journey with millions of others who are facing the realities of Alzheimer's disease. It is from this perspective that this book is written. We are not experts in the field. No one in our family is a trained medical professional or counselor. We are a very ordinary family who never expected to be where we've found ourselves over the last three years. My aunt is 76 years old and she is currently battling the effects of the disease. Some days with her are great and others are very difficult. As we are learning how to handle the situations resulting from Alzheimer's, we have been privileged to meet some amazing friends who are on the same journey. Some of our new friends have the disease. Others are the family members and caregivers. One thing is certain. Alzheimer's is devastating and dealing with it puts a family on a roller coaster of emotions. Many of those emotions are ugly at times. As I look back over the last three years, I see experiences that were especially difficult because we didn't know what was "normal" with this disease. Many of the struggles and heartbreaks might have been avoided had we been better informed from the beginning. While I don't know all the scientific explanations of Alzheimer's, I do know the pain. Our family is still experiencing that pain and I've watched other families on a daily basis as they struggle, too. I hope that sharing our story and struggles will help other families in the same situation.

1 All the statistics included in this paragraph are from the Alzheimer's Association's website (www. alz.org).

ALZHEIMER'S: Where Do We Go From Here?

CHAPTER 2

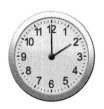

Getting A Diagnosis

ALZHEIMER'S: Where Do We Go From Here?

CHAPTER 2

Getting A Diagnosis

Once you begin to notice changes in your loved one's behavior it is difficult to know what to do next. I suppose the natural tendency is to try to pretend everything's okay or to blame the changes on the normal aging process. We first saw changes in my Aunt Betty (not her real name) about a year before she was diagnosed with Alzheimer's. Mom and Aunt Betty usually talked on the phone two or three times a week. My mother was approaching one of those "major milestone" birthdays and Aunt Betty kept asking her over and over again how old she would be on her birthday. At first, Aunt Betty asked often but in different conversations. Then it was once in every conversation. Gradually, she began asking two or three times within the same phone call. We didn't understand why she was so obsessed with Mom's age. She knew her own age and that Mom was fourteen years younger. Why couldn't she simply do the math to determine Mom's age? We now realize it was because she couldn't remember. With time, the phone conversations became more and more confusing and questions were repeated about other topics, too. Mom found it extremely frustrating to try to carry on a conversation and would often hang up after a call and say, "Good Grief. Trying to talk to her on the phone is a real challenge!" The challenge grew as time passed. In retrospect, it is easy to see what was happening though we did not understand at the time. Aunt Betty had never been one to listen carefully. We thought she was not paying attention and that was one reason for her confusion. Although she never discussed it, Aunt Betty must have been aware that she was having a problem. When we moved her close to us, we found information in her home that she had requested from the Alzheimer's Association.

Along with the confusion came increased anger. Aunt Betty had been married for 45 years. During her marriage, my uncle had been unfaithful. She had lived many years with the embarrassment and hurt caused by his infidelity. Those closest to her were always aware of her situation, but she never wanted anyone else to know. She had grown up with the idea of "not airing one's dirty laundry in public." To admit the truth would only increase the pain and embarrassment. However, during the year that preceded the diagnosis, Aunt Betty became consumed with an intense hatred toward her husband. It was impossible to keep her focused for very long on anything other than her hatred for him. Every phone conversation or visit revolved around this topic. Every time he drove out of the driveway, she was convinced he was headed to meet one of his women. She grew to despise the sight of him. Profanity and bitterness spewed from her mouth at the mere mention of his name. She no longer cared who knew her secrets and reacted with the same animosity both publicly and privately. We tried to explain to her that there was no way he was doing all she suspected. After all, he was a 70 year old man with some serious physical problems of his own. No matter how much we tried reasoning with her, she just couldn't let go of her suspicions. It was difficult to know what to do to help her. The distance between our homes and Aunt Betty's home only complicated the situation as we recognized the changes in her behavior but never considered the possibility of Alzheimer's. We understood that there was a history of infidelity and, therefore, some justification to her suspicions. What we didn't understand was the change in her attitude and behavior regarding this situation. My uncle swore that while it was true he had been unfaithful in the past, he was no longer doing any of the things my aunt suspected. In spite of this, it did sometimes seem that he deliberately tried to make her suspicious in an effort to torment her.

She had talked about filing for divorce many times through the years, but she never did anything about it. Suddenly, she decided to go through with it and divorce proceedings were begun. She was still capable of understanding that a divorce meant she and Uncle John (not his real name either) would have to sell all they owned and divide their assets. This only added to her hatred for him. She became convinced that he was slowly stealing all she owned. We felt that some time away from him would help her see life more clearly. We invited her to come for a short visit. She refused our repeated invitations because she believed he'd take another woman into her home while she was away. She feared that there'd be nothing left when she returned. As the situation deteriorated, friends and family started avoiding Aunt Betty. She acquired the reputation of being out of control. We now understand that the change in attitude and the increased anger were probably the result of Alzheimer's. Suspicion, which is sometimes a symptom of Alzheimer's disease, contributed to the years of unresolved pain to create a volatile situation.

Confusion, forgetfulness, and isolation led Aunt Betty to a place of extreme vulnerability. She spent most of her time alone at home watching Uncle John come and go. If he was at home, he spent all his time in his shop. He came inside only at bedtime. For years, he'd had a problem with alcohol. He always did his drinking late in the afternoon and early evenings. By bedtime, he was mellowed out and went to bed immediately once he came into the house. Aunt Betty was starved for love and companionship. Unfortunately, a distant family member became aware of her vulnerability and loneliness. For the last 30 years he had spent little time with Aunt Betty and had never had a close relationship with her. Suddenly he started coming to see her. Before long, he was coming three or four times a week. He hugged and kissed Aunt Betty and told her how much he loved her. As a result, Aunt Betty's money began to disappear. We feel that he took advantage of her. If questioned about it now, Aunt Betty is still adamant that she asked him to hide the money for her so that her husband would not get it. She insists she never gave him anything to keep for himself. He admits this was the case, and yet he refuses to give the money back because he says she does not need it. After checking her financial records, we realized the amount of money missing exceeds $140,000. Knowing how worried she was about having enough to live on once her divorce was completed, it is impossible to believe she consciously chose to give away that much money.

Unfortunately, the deception did not end there. Another family member entered the picture with equally questionable motives. He arrived at Aunt Betty's home on the day that Uncle John died and announced that he had come to stay for as long as was necessary. Since he was not working at that time, he was available to stay. We lived over 1500 miles away and he lived less than 200 miles from Aunt Betty. Commuting back and forth was much easier and less expensive for him. In addition, Uncle John had already hired and paid caregivers in advance to stay with Aunt Betty. Mom made plans to return to Aunt Betty's home within five or six weeks and this was openly discussed. Family members and others were aware of these plans all along. In the meantime, Mom and I called Aunt Betty daily to check on her condition and we began looking for an assisted living facility close to our homes. We realized that a memory care facility might become necessary in the future. During the daily phone calls, Mom questioned the family member often about expenses he might be incurring and offered several times to reimburse him. Each time he responded that they could take care of that later. Without our knowledge, he filed for guardianship of Aunt Betty. He was aware of the legal documents giving my mother and me authority to act as Aunt Betty's Medical and Durable Power of Attorney. When later questioned by the court-appointed guardian ad litem, Aunt Betty was able to clearly state her wishes for Mom and me to act on her behalf. We believe the family member was attempting to present a false picture to the court portraying us as having deserted Aunt Betty while he was the one who had come to her rescue. He went to the small town bank where Aunt Betty conducted her business and attempted to get into her accounts. The bank manager knew my aunt well and was aware of her desire for Mom to act as her Power of Attorney. She denied access to Aunt Betty's accounts to this other person. Once the guardian ad litem saw the legal documents and questioned Aunt Betty as to her wishes, he informed the family member that he had no basis for his case.

Why am I including all these sordid details in a book about Alzheimer's disease? Alzheimer's is horrible enough without extenuating circumstances such as these. For our family, the pain has been made many times greater because of having to deal with all the ugly issues occurring on the sidelines. If you suspect that someone you love might have Alzheimer's or another form of dementia, do whatever is necessary to protect her and her wishes. If she is still coherent enough to make sound decisions, help her see that all her paperwork is in order. Ask if she has legal documents that state who she would want to make decisions on her behalf should she become unable to do so. Since this will usually be one's spouse, ask if a second person is mentioned in case the spouse is no longer living or is unable to act in such a capacity. Be certain that those mentioned as the responsible parties have physical possession or know the exact location of all originals of the legal documentation. If these papers are stored, it is crucial that they are in a safe place, such as a safe deposit box in a bank, where access is limited. This may seem unnecessary, but the unfortunate reality is that money tends to bring out the worst in some people. Our family's experiences are not unique. We've met others who've had similar challenges. Having a copy of such documentation is sufficient in some states while the original is necessary in others. Protecting your loved one's wishes is a very important aspect of dealing with the disease.

ALZHEIMER'S: Where Do We Go From Here?

Sixteen months ago my aunt began to experience severe stomach pain. After three trips to the hospital, an accurate diagnosis was finally made. Emergency surgery followed. She remained in the hospital for one week after the surgery. Once she was released from the hospital, she went to a rehab facility for one month. Three weeks after she returned home, Uncle John died from a self-inflicted gunshot wound. Five weeks later she was taken to a care facility to live. We brought her to live in a center near our homes after two weeks in the first facility. Aunt Betty went from living independently at home, driving around town, and taking no medication to living in a facility and being on a long list of medications within a four-month period. We have been told that, most likely, the onset of the disease was greatly escalated by the physical trauma of the surgery and anesthesia and the emotional trauma of Uncle John's death. Fortunately, Alzheimer's doesn't come on that quickly in all cases.

As we've compared stories with other Alzheimer's families, it has been interesting to learn what they first noticed that led them to consider Alzheimer's as the cause. A friend's family had two people with the disease. Both of those folks first began having difficulty performing simple math problems. Another woman suddenly began preparing very easy meals that required little memory instead of the big meals she had always prepared in the past. One person had several minor car accidents and even drove off from one accident without realizing what she was doing. Forgetfulness was common in every case. One lady went to the wrong bank. Another would frequently go into her favorite restaurant and order food to go. Before it was ready, she'd forget and leave without her order. Others began repeating things. Someone else parked her car in a lot and could not find it later because she had forgotten what kind of car she had. A man whose job required him to do technical writing became insecure about his work and had someone proofread everything he wrote. One lady became fearful at night. Others became confused about directions and got lost when driving within their own neighborhoods. Several began driving recklessly. A friend's mother became very insecure about her money and was obsessed with having her purse close to her at all times. Some Alzheimer's victims became reclusive and never wanted to leave home. Difficulty communicating was an early symptom for others. Though these strange things occurred, all these people acted "normal" in other ways. That's one of the most bizarre parts of Alzheimer's.

I've heard it said that only hindsight is 20/20. Looking back it is easy to see a pattern of behaviors prior to my aunt's diagnosis. If we could go back and relive that time again, we'd do many things differently. We now have an idea of where to begin. First, check out the internet for any resources you can find pertaining to Alzheimer's. Then contact any organizations such as the Alzheimer's Association for information about symptoms, diagnosis, treatment, etc. Visit your local library. Inquire at your local city or county health department about any information they might have available. Plan a visit to the doctor without your family member to discuss your concerns and get advice from him. Laws protecting patient privacy always need to be respected, but the originals of the Medical Power of Attorney will make it easier for those named in the document to gain access to the doctor. If the doctor is a general practitioner, ask for a referral to a geriatric specialist who deals specifically with Alzheimer's. Ask questions about how to handle the situation. Do you tell your loved one you suspect a problem? How do you get them to a doctor to be tested without upsetting them? This is the kind of information that you need to know before your loved one ever sees a doctor. I know families who have told their loved one he/she had Alzheimer's. Others were advised not to tell because the victim will often turn on the ones who give him that information. Advice from experts in the field will help you know how to proceed. Locate an Alzheimer's support group and make it a priority to attend their meetings. Such groups are usually led by a trained medical and/or mental health professional knowledgeable of the various aspects of Alzheimer's. You might discover that the members of a support group have already dealt with the issues you are facing. They may be able to provide a wealth of information and encouragement as ones who've "been there and done that," especially those who are dealing with the latter stages of the disease. They understand the emotional aspect of facing the disease personally. All these resources can help to determine if Alzheimer's is an accurate diagnosis and what to do next.

ALZHEIMER'S: Where Do We Go From Here?

CHAPTER 3

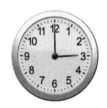

Home Care VS
A Specialized Facility

CHAPTER 3

Home Care VS A Specialized Facility

One of the most difficult aspects of caring for someone with Alzheimer's is the decision concerning where the person will reside. Obviously, trained professionals would have more insight into this area. They can speak from a much greater base of experience and knowledge. They should know the various stages of the disease and have an idea of what to expect as the disease progresses. A determination of whether home or a specialized care facility is the best option should include the advice of those trained to deal with Alzheimer's.

Since each person is unique and family situations vary, it seems a broad definitive answer to this dilemma might be difficult or even impossible. One major consideration is how far advanced the disease is. If it's more advanced, more care is required. Do other medical problems also exist? Who is at home to care for the Alzheimer's patient? How will the family be impacted by a decision to remain at home? Will someone be available to stay with the person 24 hours a day? Who can relieve the primary caregiver?

Do financial resources allow for the person to move into an acceptable care facility? Is there an acceptable facility in the area? Will the Alzheimer's victim have a higher quality of life at home or in a care facility? These questions must be answered before a decision can be made.

We know families who decided to keep their loved one at home during the first stages of the disease, but later moved them into a facility. They eventually realized they had waited too long before moving them. Their reason was that the rest of their family was neglected because they were so consumed with the care of the one with Alzheimer's who was not even aware of his surroundings. In addition, they felt that they were required to give up too much of their own lives. To someone who has never experienced the daily stress associated with caring for an Alzheimer's sufferer, this may sound cruel or selfish. Those of us who have dealt with the demands firsthand understand that sometimes a facility is the best option. However, realizing it may be best does not eliminate the heartache of moving someone you love into such a place.

For our family's experience, someone else left Aunt Betty at a care facility before we were notified. We received a call in which a family member informed us that it had become necessary to take her to a facility for physical therapy. The facility happened to be a memory care unit. We were told that we should not call or visit for two weeks. We found the story to be somewhat suspicious. When we contacted the memory care unit and questioned why it was necessary to have no contact with her for the two-week period, they informed us this information was incorrect. We believe that was part of the plan to make it appear that we'd deserted Aunt Betty. When we arrived at the facility we found her so heavily over-medicated she could not stand, go to the bathroom, or eat without help. Obviously, her memory was impaired by too much medicine as well. She has no recollection of how she came to reside in our town or of her time in the other facility. Once we moved her to her current residence and her medications were reduced, she was so happy to be near our family that she accepted the new surroundings surprisingly well. There have been times when she wanted to look for an apartment or house, but overall she has been very satisfied in the Center. Since we had no other option, we are very thankful that she has been so content in her new home.

Staying at home (either the home of the person with Alzheimer's or the home of a family member) has some advantages. The Alzheimer's sufferer will feel more comfortable with the familiar surroundings of home. If the spouse is still living, the couple will be able to continue living together. Staying at home also provides a certain feeling of "normalcy" for the family at the onset of the disease. Unless an outside caregiver is employed, no additional expense is involved. We've all heard those horror stories about nursing homes and abuse of the elderly. As a result, some families might feel more at ease with care being provided by a loved one rather than strangers.

Some of the disadvantages of staying at home may outweigh the benefits. For instance, 24-hour care is exhausting for those responsible for the Alzheimer's patient. A spouse cannot continue looking after their mate indefinitely. As the disease progresses, the sufferer must be watched carefully every time he moves. Will he turn on the stove or start to fill the bathtub and walk away, forgetting what he just did? Will he wander away from home? If he finds car keys, will he drive away in the car? Will he become agitated and be too much for the caregiver to handle? Will the caregiver be able to bathe and dress him once he is no longer able to do so alone? Who will help with issues related to incontinence? When his sleep patterns are no longer normal, how long will the caregiver be able to stay awake with him? If outside caregivers become necessary, where will the family find dependable workers? Will the cost of three shifts per day exceed the cost of a facility? These are only a few of the problems that must be addressed if the decision is made for the Alzheimer's victim to remain at home.

Once the person with Alzheimer's reaches the point where he requires more help than can be provided at home, a care facility becomes necessary. Admitting this is painful. I imagine it's the hardest of all for a spouse to relocate the one they love to a separate residence. Locating an acceptable place is not easy, but there are advantages to moving your loved one into a specialized home. The most obvious benefit is that the family has less responsibility for 24-hour care of the one with the disease. The physical, mental, and emotional demands are lessened. The staff of a memory care facility will be trained to handle the effects of the disease. The person suffering with Alzheimer's has an opportunity to socialize with others who are usually close to his same age and who also share his same frustrations. Depending on the individual facility, the person might feel he has more independence than if he lived with a family member other than his spouse. The care facility can offer activities that provide the kind of stimulation an Alzheimer's patient needs. A center should be able to provide a more structured environment and schedule and, therefore, promote feelings of security for the residents. Some specialized facilities have Registered Nurses on the premises around the clock. Immediate medical help is important for a person with Alzheimer's.

On the other hand, disadvantages should also be examined before moving your loved one into a care center. Cost is a major consideration. The rules for Medicare and Medicaid are complicated for these types of residences. Every place is unique. Some are excellent and others are not. Can you really trust the staff to treat your loved one well once you leave? Sharing a bedroom is usually necessary and even encouraged at many facilities. One advantage to sharing is the mental stimulation of having to interact with someone else. The cost will be less for a shared room than for a private one. However, it might be a difficult adjustment for some people to share a room with a stranger. Residents tend to wander in and out of each other's rooms and personal belongings sometimes disappear. Finally, an unfortunate reality is that employees might sometimes steal from the residents, too.

As we've met many family members of Alzheimer's victims and heard their stories, I've been curious to hear when and why they finally moved their loved one into a facility. Most did so only because they felt they had no other choice. One family moved their mother in once it became apparent that she was very near death. They did not want her to die at home. Others did so because they knew the person with the disease would be happier with some "life" around her instead of sitting at home with an outside caregiver day after day. Regardless of the reason, it's always a tough decision and is usually harder for the family than for the Alzheimer's victim.

We've discovered that many places allow respite care for a few days at a time. This is an option for families who are not ready to move the Alzheimer's sufferer in permanently. The primary caregiver gets a break for a few days or weeks while their loved one stays in a facility. Another idea is to have someone stay in a center only during the day as opposed to full time. A third option is to take your family member in two or three days per week to allow him time for interaction with others who are dealing with his same struggles. The rest of the time could be spent at home with the help of paid caregivers outside of the family. Either of these options might be an easier transition into living full time in a specialized care facility.

It is important to note that not all facilities are created equal. I remember as a young girl going to visit my great grandmother in a nursing home. The awful stench of urine still comes to my mind 30 years later. I remember the agonizing cries of residents who had fallen out of their chairs and were left lying on the floor. Worst of all, I remember entering my great grandmother's room on many occasions and finding her clothes and bedding caked with dried feces that had been ignored and the sores that resulted. She wasn't in a bad nursing home. Supposedly, she was in one of the good ones. Now I understand that not all nursing homes and care facilities are like that one, but some are.

When we began searching for a place for Aunt Betty, we discovered that three types of specialized care facilities existed:

(1) assisted living with a memory care unit,
(2) nursing homes, and
(3) facilities entirely devoted to memory care.

I was horrified by the first facility we visited. We were first given a tour of the assisted living area. Each resident had two private rooms complete with a large bathroom and kitchenette. We were shown the activities room filled with games, puzzles, and craft supplies and a bright, cheerfully decorated ice cream parlor. There were several beautifully furnished common areas for visiting with other residents and guests. An in-house beauty shop provided residents with yet another convenience. Our tour of this area was completed with a peek into two elegant dining areas. Residents were free to come and go and the large parking lot had ample spaces for each one's car. We thought, "What a wonderful place! Aunt Betty would be so happy living here!" Then reality stepped in. "So, would you like to see our memory care area now?" asked the woman who was giving us the tour. The scene quickly changed from pleasant to horrific. The excitement and hope we were feeling was quickly replaced by disappointment and fear. The smell of urine permeated into the hallway from beneath the heavy, metal locked door. We felt as if we were entering a prison when we stepped through the doorway. Residents were aimlessly wandering back and forth around a very small living area. Our attention was directed to two dining rooms. One was for residents who could no longer feed themselves and the other was for those who could still eat without help. The woman wanted us to see how the more independent residents were able to watch each other and mirror the actions necessary to feed themselves, even if it was with their hands instead of utensils. Mom, Leigh, and I were all emotional as we exited the building. We sat in the car and discussed how difficult it will be if Aunt Betty's condition should progress to that of many of the residents in that particular place.

As we visited other assisted living centers and nursing homes in our area, this scenario was repeated over and over. All the assisted living centers were attractive and inviting upon entry. Most were decorated with elaborate brass chandeliers and lovely Queen Anne style furniture. They were all the types of places that most people would be proud to call home. However, we were always directed to a back building or hall where those suffering from Alzheimer's and dementia resided. Needless to say, those places never looked the same as the rest of the building. They all resembled the memory care unit of the first place we had visited. We always left feeling disappointed. The nursing homes we visited were all very hospital-like and depressing. Aunt Betty is still coherent about most things. How could we ever move her into any of these places and have her aware of the conditions around her? She would feel like she had been imprisoned. We knew we could not do that to her. She needed to be in a place where she could make friends and converse with people around her. She needed emotional and mental stimulation and room to roam around in a safe atmosphere. Did such a place exist? For our family, we know that God directed us to the Center where Aunt Betty now lives.

When we entered, we were delighted to see French doors with windows so the residents could see outside. To ensure no one wanders off, the exterior doors are locked and regulated by a keypad adjacent to the doors. A staff member is usually nearby to redirect the residents away from these doors. This was much more pleasant than the heavy solid one we had first experienced. There is a large common area where residents are free to play games, eat, visit with friends and family, take a nap, relax on a sofa or recliner, or enjoy special entertainment. A tall wrought iron fence surrounds the property so residents are free to roam outside within safe confines. A large gazebo and several awnings provide great places to sit and enjoy fresh air and sunshine. Each of the four wings of the building has a large TV and a comfortable sitting area. The philosophy of the Center is to allow residents as much independence as possible. We left after that first visit confident that we'd finally located the right place. The Center is not perfect, but we do believe it is one of the best. Since that day we've learned that a facility is only as good as the staff, regardless of how beautiful it may be. We have been extremely blessed to have wonderful care given by people who genuinely love my aunt. We will be forever indebted to them for all they've done to help Aunt Betty and our family. They treat all the residents with dignity and respect and work to provide them a home, not an institution.

After spending a year and a half visiting the Center on a regular basis, I now realize that the horror we felt in that first place was not because of the condition of the residents but because of the conditions in which they lived. They were locked up behind that awful door in a tight, dark, dreary portion of the building that represented captivity while all the residents on the other side of the door enjoyed freedom. It was as if those who had been victimized by Alzheimer's were being treated like little caged animals. I hope I never have to go inside another place like that again. Fortunately, there are good places for your loved ones with Alzheimer's. It may take some time and searching, but we know they do exist. Don't give up until you feel comfortable with your choice, but be prepared for some unpleasant visits while you search for the right place.

Once you find a place you feel is satisfactory, stay on top of all that's happening. Visit often and during different shifts. Get to know the staff. Question anything that bothers you. Pay attention to changes in your loved one. If you notice something different, ask if there have been any changes in medicine. Sometimes these changes are the result of the disease and other times they may be caused by a particular medicine. Don't be afraid to stand up for your loved one who can't stand up for himself. Remember, he's counting on you, whether at home or in a facility.

ALZHEIMER'S: Where Do We Go From Here?

CHAPTER 4

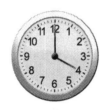

A Few Of My
Favorite Things

ALZHEIMER'S: Where Do We Go From Here?

CHAPTER 4

A Few Of My Favorite Things

We all have things that we enjoy. Most of the time we take the simple pleasures of everyday life for granted. For the person with Alzheimer's, these pleasures take on greater significance. For the past year I've watched the people who reside in the same memory care facility as my aunt to see what seems to bring them the most pleasure. I've been amazed at how simple most of these things are.

My aunt and her roommate have birthdays that fall within two weeks of each other. Last year we had a big party for the two of them. Both families got together and carried the birthday girls out to lunch at a nearby restaurant. We had a private dining room reserved especially for us. Since our girls were turning 76 and 77, we decided to decorate the room with a "Red Hat Society" theme. For those of you who are not familiar with the Red Hat Society, it is made up of groups of women who are all 55 years old or older. They have no special agenda for anything other than fun. To identify themselves, the group members will usually wear red or purple clothing with a big red and purple hat. All the women at our party wore red hats, too. Everyone enjoyed the day, but the birthday girls enjoyed it the most. They were both so cute posing for pictures in their hats and opening all their gifts. They "oohed" and "aahed" over every package. Since each of them loves tomatoes, we put together two small baskets with two big, juicy tomatoes. When they opened their baskets, they cried. With all the nice gifts they received, they cried over a couple of tomatoes. Why? Those tomatoes represented an act of kindness to them. My mom and I had gone out of town for three days about two weeks before the party. During that time, Dad stopped by each day with tomatoes and fresh bread for our girls. He made them sandwiches and hot coffee. They had enjoyed the attention and talked about how sweet it was for him to think of them after he had worked all day. That's why they both cried when they opened their baskets. Dad's thoughtful deed had made them feel special. When they returned from their party, all the pretty new clothes were put away and the sink counter in the bathroom was lined with tomatoes. They were proud of those tomatoes and shed even more tears over the next few days whenever they thought about them. I realized that day how big the little things can be in someone's life, especially if it's someone who has already lost so much to Alzheimer's.

Tomatoes aren't the only food that our girls enjoy. We often carry them chocolate, BLT sandwiches, chicken salad, chili dogs, ice cream sundaes, and anything else they may mention wanting. I often notice other residents enjoying special treats their families have brought to them, too. When you're no longer able to go out and get what you like, it's important that someone else remembers and does that for you.

One of my aunt's new friends gets fresh flowers delivered to her every few days. Her sister, who lives in another state, is unable to visit her so she sends her flowers. A beautiful fresh floral arrangement makes her room look pretty and smell great, in addition to reminding her that someone loves her.

Many of those who reside in the Center still love to dance. The activities staff makes certain that the schedule is filled with music of all kinds. Sometimes the residents enjoy tunes from the 1940's and other times the place may sound more like a honky-tonk with a country and western flavor. Then there are occasions when a pianist serenades them with old hymns or a flutist plays more classical arrangements. Regardless of the musical style, the residents always respond positively. If there's music, there's usually dancing. The daughter of one resident will come whenever special music is on the calendar. She and her mother dance around the large gathering room together. Her mother always has a huge smile as she dances. It's obvious that she's never lost her love for dancing and that this simple act of love from her daughter brings her great joy. Since so many others also enjoy dancing, some of the staff members will usually partner up with them. The footwork may not be as impressive as it once was, but the pleasure it gives is heartwarming to see.

Another resident is an avid dominoes player. She walks around with her dominoes in her bag at all times and is always ready to take on a new opponent. She seldom loses a game. One day I overheard a conversation between my teenaged daughter and this woman during one of their games. My daughter informed her that she needed to stop playing because we had to leave but that she'd play dominoes with her again when she returned the next day. The lady asked if she promised she'd do that. My daughter promised. Then I heard this woman say, "I love you" to my daughter as a smile covered her face. Again, this was an example of something small that was a big deal in someone's life that day.

One of the male residents has always been a big fan of golf. The Center has a putter and a few golf balls along with a small putting green with three holes. Our friend can be found most days with the bucket of balls and putter in his hands headed to the "golf course." Sometimes his brother comes and plays with him. When they finish their game, I enjoy asking him how he played. He compares his playing to Arnold Palmer's and we usually laugh. Golf is still one of his favorite pastimes. The lush, green courses of the past have been replaced by a single Astroturf putting green, but the pleasure of the game remains.

My aunt has always cared about her appearance. She has enjoyed having pretty clothes and feeling like her hair and makeup looked good. Manicured nails were important to her, too. Now that we are responsible for her care, we make her appearance a priority. We take her shopping and help her find things that she likes. Even when she's had trouble walking or standing due to her osteoporosis, she's been able to get into a department store fitting room to try on clothes. We have to hold on tightly to her to keep her from falling, but she still manages to get in front of a mirror and model for us. She loves strutting, as she calls it, up and down the halls of the Center while wearing a new outfit. She still goes to the beauty salon once a week to have her hair done. We carry her to the nail salon and she gets pedicures and manicures. When she walks back into the Center upon her return, she has to stop and show her hands to everyone she passes. The caregivers call her "the Princess" because she always looks so nice and she thrives on the attention. Knowing how much pleasure she receives from this attention, how could we do anything less than keep her looking and feeling good?

Along with her personal appearance, my aunt has always cared about the appearance of her surroundings. Since moving her to the memory care facility, we've attempted to make her room as attractive as possible.

We carried in some of her personal belongings to make it feel more like home. She has a curio cabinet filled with special knick knacks that remind her of happy times in the past. There are pictures of family, too. Over her bed hangs an 11 x 14 picture of my grandparents. When she sits in her recliner, she can see their picture. She seems to find comfort from it. She and her roommate each have a telephone with a list of phone numbers. Feeling that they can reach us whenever they want is also a source of comfort to them. They have a TV in their room and even though they can't always follow the storyline of the programs, it provides good background noise when they're in the room. Having their own TV makes their room seem more like home, too.

Many of the residents love to see young children come to visit. The Center is rather unique because the employees are allowed to bring their children to work with them. It's fun to watch the older folks' faces brighten when they see these young visitors. One little boy has always come to work with his mother. Three-year-old Anthony has big, brown eyes that sparkle. Anthony regularly brings joy to the lives of the residents.

Another unusual part of the home is that they allow pets. There are three dogs owned by the Center and currently one resident has her own dog. In addition, two residents have cats. Three large bird cages are filled with various birds. These animals are a source of pleasure for the residents. It's interesting to see how much comfort and security can be gained from holding a cuddly little animal on one's lap.

These are just a few of the things that can turn a sad, lonely day into a good one for someone with Alzheimer's. The list of suggestions is infinite. For one precious woman, it's as simple as the color red. She loves red, whether that's red shoes, nails, or clothes. My point is to help you start thinking about your loved one and trying to come up with ways to brighten a day. As you can see from these examples, it's usually the smallest, simplest things that bring the greatest pleasure. Taking the time to do these things for your loved one will add quality to her life and give you special moments with her that will be cherished in the days ahead.

ALZHEIMER'S: Where Do We Go From Here?

CHAPTER 5

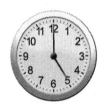

Everybody's Doing It

CHAPTER 5

Everybody's Doing It

U nderstanding a few of the similarities that exist among Alzheimer's patients may spare the family from some of the emotional pain. Realizing that everybody else is doing the same thing makes it much easier to deal with some of the behaviors your loved one may exhibit from time to time. It's not easy to find yourself in charge of another person's life. Many of the decisions are heart-wrenching. Even though Aunt Betty had already been moved into a facility by another relative without our knowledge, we still struggled with the choice we were forced to make once we began making decisions on her behalf. We feel that we rescued her from a miserable situation when we moved her into a memory care residence close to us. As I've mentioned before, she was so heavily medicated in the first place that she has no recollection of ever being there. Still, we agonized over certain aspects of her transition to the new environment. She said and did things that made us feel an enormous guilt. For the entire first year, we only missed five or six days of visiting her. Some days only one or two of us were with Aunt Betty, but many days she was visited by my mother, daughter and me. For each visit we stayed for three or four hours. She was the most-often visited resident in the home. We tried our best to ensure that she never felt sad or lonely if we could help it. Gradually, we started to realize that the same things Aunt Betty was doing were being repeated by almost every other resident in the home. Her behaviors were really quite typical of an Alzheimer's patient, or at least they are typical of the approximately 100 people who we've been observing for more than a year. We had no reason to feel any guilt. We are in no way responsible for any sadness she feels. The disease gets all the blame. This realization was like having a huge burden lifted from our shoulders.

Aunt Betty often talks about her mother and asks if she is still alive. At times she wants us to take her home so she can check on her. She asks us when we've spoken to her or when we've last seen her. She grieves for her mother. My grandmother passed away nearly 25 years ago. Aunt Betty was there, made all the funeral arrangements, and even served as executor of her estate. Yet, she has so much trouble remembering that Grandmother is no longer living. Sometimes when she does remember, she thinks it has just happened so she grieves as if she has just learned of the news. We thought that she was struggling with this because of the unusually close relationship she and my grandmother shared and that her behavior was unique to her. One day I realized that three other residents were also looking for their mothers. One woman was looking for her father. A couple of others were waiting for their deceased husbands to pick them up. Looking for someone who is no longer living is not at all unusual in this setting. They may not remember that their spouse has already passed away so it's easy to see why they wait for them to come. Since Alzheimer's sufferers tend to revert back to an earlier time in life, such as childhood, it's also somewhat "normal" for them to look for their parents.

Most of the time, Aunt Betty is content in her new surroundings. However, she occasionally decides that she needs to go home. She has never wanted to go back to her home to live, but she has wanted to go home long enough to sell the house so she can buy a new place in our city. For a while she talked about her own place. With time we noticed that "home" had shifted from her house to my grandparents' house. She became obsessed with the need to sell it. She could not remember that she sold it more than 25 years ago.

In over 16 months I've never heard one woman say anything except, "I want to go home." She walks around and repeats that over and over again day after day. Another dear lady often asks if we know the way to the bus station so she can get home. On one particular day we told her that we were unaware of a bus station in the area. She responded that she thought she would ride her bike instead. Knowing her prim personality, we thought this reaction was a bit comical. Wanting to go home is another familiar part of Alzheimer's for residents who have moved into a care facility. It could be a negative reflection on the place, but our experience has shown that it is probably due to the common behaviors of this disease.

Around 4:00 each afternoon you can see a change take place in the general mood of many Alzheimer's patients. This change is called "sundowning". I don't know all the medical explanations of what's occurring, but I've watched enough folks to realize this is most likely to be the time of day when one might become more confused, depressed, or agitated. This seems to be the most difficult time to end a visit because Aunt Betty will usually start to cry when we leave. In the last few months we've noticed another change in Aunt Betty. If we take her out for a while, she starts wanting to go back around 4:00. She needs the security of the Center. If we stay and eat with her, she is no longer comfortable eating in another dining room other than her usual one. Several times she has gotten up from the table with us, walked back to her regular spot in her dining room, and left us sitting in another room. The familiarity of doing the same thing at the same place is especially important once she begins sundowning.

I know of an Alzheimer's victim who still lives at home with his wife. He is so worried about his car keys that he sleeps with them under his pillow. I was told that he awakens during the night and pulls the keys out to make sure they're still there. It is not unusual to find one of our friends with Alzheimer's looking for keys or other personal items. We bought a small wrist-sized coil that Aunt Betty can wear on her arm like a bracelet so her keys are always in sight and easily accessible. Many of the other residents have similar bands or neck lanyards for their keys. This seems to give them a little peace of mind. Aunt Betty was so upset about not being able to find her car keys that we put together a ring of old keys for her. She's never realized they are not really her keys. She keeps them in her purse and that gives her a sense of comfort. Lost purses can also create havoc for the residents as they frantically search for them. My aunt often becomes anxious because she is unable to locate her checkbook. We finally had to put some deposit slips in her checkbook cover so she would feel calmer when she opened her purse to find checks. Obviously, we can't put her real checks in her purse, including those for a closed-out account because of the risk of identity theft. The manager of the bank warned us of putting in anything other than generic deposit slips. Alzheimer's patients also tend to worry about their cars. It is a common occurrence to find one of the residents pacing from door to door looking for his car in the parking lot. We learned of one family that drove the car of the resident to the home and parked it in the lot so their loved one would feel more satisfied when she looked out and saw her car in the lot. Any time they took her out of the home, they drove her car. This is probably not practical for most families, but for this one it brought comfort to the resident.

As I've mentioned before, some people with Alzheimer's experience a drastic change in personality. Some become more passive and others become more assertive. I've noticed that even the most passive ones can become defiant at times. It's interesting to see what triggers a refusal to cooperate. For my aunt, it is taking her medicine. She takes several medications throughout the day. Most of the time, she willingly swallows the medicine without any objections. However, she sometimes reasons that she's never taken much medicine in her life and she's not going to start now. Any attempt to convince her otherwise will only end in an angry episode. We've found that if she is left alone for five or ten minutes she will usually take them upon a second attempt. A few days ago I watched one of the residents who is a kind, extremely polite, gentle person pinch one of the caregivers who was trying to convince him to go to his dining room for lunch. I've never seen him do anything like that before, but at that moment he definitely refused to cooperate. He wanted to stay in another room with a group who had gathered for a private party. Once they persuaded him that they'd call him if they needed him, he calmed down and peacefully walked to his regular dining area.

For some of the residents, tears are a part of daily life. My heart goes out to some of them because they seem so lost and afraid. One little woman comes to my mind. I think her family lives a long distance from the home so she seldom has visitors. Each time we walk past her she reaches out for our hands. She grabs hold to us as if she were reaching for a lifeline. Tears gently roll down her cheeks as she asks if she's bothering us. Another woman who has a much stronger personality often spots one of us when we enter the home. She hurriedly rolls her wheelchair to meet us. She usually grabs our hands and begins mumbling something to us. These encounters tend to end with her head in her lap and tears streaming down her face. My aunt has frequent crying spells, too. Generally, they last only a few minutes and they most often occur because she has remembered my grandmother. She does sometimes have days when she cries about everything. If anyone is kind to her, she cries. If someone says something that hurts her feelings, she cries. Almost anything will set off a flood of tears. Her roommate has days like this, too. Things that would not bother her most days will produce a bucket of tears on other days. Both my aunt and her roommate are strong women, but their emotional systems seem to be so weakened by their disease that they sometimes appear more fragile than usual. Other patients exhibit similar characteristics.

Since people suffering with Alzheimer's tend to revert back to an earlier time, it is commonplace to hear them referring to the home as their school, or to the dining room as their classroom, or to the administrator as their principal. We've heard them describing each other as classmates and the staff as secretary or president of their class. The home has entertainment on a regular basis and these get-togethers are often referred to by the residents as classes in school. Naturally, it follows that the large gathering room must be the school auditorium. At these times, it is obvious that the person has mentally returned to his childhood.

Another curious similarity we've noticed among the residents is an inability to accurately perceive their surroundings. The home where my aunt lives is a large one-story building shaped like an "H" with four different wings of bedrooms and a huge common area in the middle. Most of the residents are convinced that there are at least two floors. They describe the wings where the bedrooms are located as the upstairs and the common area as the downstairs. One day we went to visit my aunt and she and her roommate were having a somewhat heated discussion about whether there were two or three floors in the home. While they couldn't agree if there were two or three, they were both certain it was more than one. I don't understand what makes them feel there is more than one floor, but it seems that many of the residents become disoriented at times regarding their surroundings.

Aggression is another problem in the home from time to time. By aggression, I mean more than the assertive-

ness I mentioned when one may refuse to take medicine or cooperate in some other way. I mean the kind of
aggression that involves hitting or pushing. We have one
friend with Alzheimer's who is a spry, spunky, pleasant
woman most of the time. If there is a resident that I would
describe as having a hyper personality, this woman would
be it. She loves to laugh and talk and is usually a lot of
fun. Nevertheless, she is quick to fight if she gets upset.
I remember a time when she hit her roommate because
she thought the roommate was sleeping in her husband's
bed. Another woman pushed three people before her
family moved her to another facility. In two of those
incidents, the person she hit sustained broken bones.
Osteoporosis is a big problem with many of these elderly
people so a simple fall or hit can often result in broken
bones. It is painful to see some of these things happen.
We realize that the one being aggressive doesn't mean to
be that way and is probably too confused to understand
the inappropriateness of his/her actions at the moment.
How can one be held responsible for something he can't
understand? On the other hand, it's not fair to allow one
person to harm others. Unfortunately, aggression seems
to be another behavior many Alzheimer's patients will
exhibit from time to time.

We've learned a new word to describe one of the
symptoms of the disease. That word is perseverating.
It means grabbing hold of a thought and not being able
to let it go. With Aunt Betty, it is usually something

related to the need to sell either her home or my grand-parent's home or discussions about how she recently lost her mother. Christmas 2005 was, in her mind, her first Christmas without my grandmother. In reality, it was her 24th. This was all she talked about for weeks before and after the holidays. She would start to talk about it and a flood of tears was always close behind. We tried over and over again to explain that her grief was making it difficult for her to remember, but she had survived 23 Christmas Days without her mom and would make it through this one, too. She remembered the year my grandmother died and she knew it was now 2005. If she would consider the fact that she would never have gone 24 years without seeing her mom, then she should be able to understand that was not her first year without her. We thought this would make her feel better. After struggling with this for weeks, one of the staff at the home told us that we were completely wrong in our approach. She told us we were trying to bring her back to reality with what we were telling her. She is incapable of understanding reality at moments such as these. Telling her the truth only caused her more frustration because she couldn't remember. The combination of frustration and grief was overwhelming for her. Perseverating on one topic or person presents a real struggle for both the Alzheimer's patient and for those who love them. Yet it seems to be a common symp-tom of the disease. We've learned that it is best in these situations to try to change the subject. My aunt is quite persistent and keeps coming back to the same topic, but we have to be more persistent than she is. Sometimes we act as if we've just remembered something we need to go do and we walk away for a minute of two. Usually this works and she will have forgotten the topic once we return. Create a distraction. That's the best way to handle perseverating.

Alzheimer's is a brutal disease. It takes its toll on the person who is diagnosed with it and all those closely involved with them. Understanding the behavioral commonalities of its victims in advance may help some families face the disease with more understanding and, therefore, less stress because you already know what to expect as "normal."

ALZHEIMER'S: Where Do We Go From Here?

CHAPTER 6

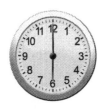

Keeping Good Records

ALZHEIMER'S: Where Do We Go From Here?

CHAPTER 6

Keeping Good Records

For many families, the amount of record keeping required for an Alzheimer's patient will be overwhelming. The information presented in this chapter is not intended to be construed as legal or financial advice. Our family consulted with a qualified attorney specializing in Estate Planning and a Certified Financial Planner to discuss our particular situation and the requirements for the state in which we live. We recommend you do the same. We are passing this information along only as a reference to the issues and advice given to our family for assistance with the care of Aunt Betty. It should not be considered appropriate for all situations. Some of the information included was gained through our personal experiences. Aunt Betty is financially stable and is not dependent on anyone else for money. The advice we have been given might not apply in a situation where a family has to provide the money for the care of their loved one. Good record keeping includes financial, legal, and medical documentation.

Alzheimer's care is expensive. The cost is directly related to the amount of care provided by people outside the family. Obviously, full-time residence in a specialized care facility can be quite expensive. However, at-home care can equal or exceed the cost of a facility if outside care is required on a 24/7 basis. Usually the amount of money available will determine which options exist regarding the care of a person with Alzheimer's. It is important to know that many facilities do not accept Medicare.

There are a few basic paperwork needs for every adult, regardless of medical or financial condition. I have already mentioned some of this information in the first chapter, but I feel a more detailed explanation is appropriate at this time. Each adult should have a Last Will and Testament that specifies his wishes for disposition of assets upon his death and for the care of any dependent children or adults. A Durable Power of Attorney will allow someone you trust to make medical and personal decisions on your behalf should you become incapacitated and unable to do so. This is important for many reasons other than Alzheimer's. An accident, heart attack, stroke, etc. could render you unable to convey your wishes to medical personnel. This could leave you at the mercy of the court system or a spouse that you may not trust, as in Aunt Betty's case, if you have not designated someone to act on your behalf. Some people do not want to put the burden of having to make life or death decisions on the shoulders of a spouse, so they choose a third party to act in this capacity. A standard Power of Attorney is essential to have someone make financial decisions and pay bills for you should you become unable to do so. It is not necessary to designate the same person or persons as the Executor of your Will and Durable and Financial Powers of Attorney. However, they need to be someone who you can trust explicitly to carry out your wishes and manage your affairs to the best of YOUR interests. As I've mentioned before, money tends to bring out the worst in some people so carefully consider your choices and discuss this with your family. It is wise to make legal decisions such as these while one is still healthy. However, once Alzheimer's is suspected or diagnosed, it is imperative these issues be resolved before it is too late.

Once the disease progresses to the point where an Alzheimer's victim is no longer considered competent, it will be too late for him to make legal decisions. If challenged in court, paperwork done for someone who is "not of sound mind" would never stand up. Most attorneys will not even attempt to handle such matters as Wills or Power of Attorney documents if they feel the person is not of sound enough mind to explicitly state his intentions and why he wants things done a certain way.

Medical care for Aunt Betty is being paid by Medicare, her Medicare Part B supplemental policy, and the Medicare Part D Prescription Drug policy. The Center has a doctor specializing in geriatric care that comes once every week to check on the residents. Family members or the Center staff can recommend or request that the doctor sees anyone during the regular visits. It is important that you keep accurate records of the visits with the doctor(s) and all medicines prescribed.

In terms of financial management, a non-Revocable Trust was recommended as the best option for Aunt Betty's money. A trust fund allows us to maintain a specific accounting of her money, how it is invested, and how it is spent. Keeping track of the cash flow is an important part of managing the often long-term and expensive care required for an Alzheimer's patient.

The cost of Alzheimer's care can be divided into two basic categories:

(1) medically necessary items and
(2) items related to quality of life.

Medically necessary items include all day-to-day care, meals, medicines, and specialized equipment such as beds, wheelchairs, walkers, etc. Quality of life items are expenses for a phone, cable TV, clothing, hair care, manicures and pedicures, and other items that provide some measure of normalcy for the person with Alzheimer's while she is still cognizant of these things. It is important to keep these two sets of expenses separate and documented accordingly. The medically necessary expenses may be deducted on income taxes while quality of life expenses are usually not deductible. This is important if there is significant investment or business income that is used to pay the expenses. You should consult with a qualified tax accountant regarding your specific situation.

Managing the finances of someone with a long-term disease can be difficult, especially if you don't start off with a good system that works for you. There is no magic method to doing this, you just need to find something that works and is easy for you to handle. There is enough stress for an Alzheimer's family without adding more because of the business end of caring for your loved one. I want to explain what we have found to be a good system for our family. Again, I stress that this is not intended to be advice to you, but only an example of one family's experiences.

The first rule of record keeping is "keep it all". Our system is relatively simple. We have a plastic three-drawer tray and a single file drawer in a desk that is dedicated to Aunt Betty's paperwork. The three drawer trays are set up for Medicare statements, Medicare Supplement statements, and Prescription Drug Plan (PDP) information. In the file drawer we have files labeled for bank statements, investment account statements, expense receipts, trust fund documents, medical documents, and a three ring binder set up for medicines. In this binder we keep track of all the medicines Aunt Betty takes. This includes name and dosage amount, what they do (a good source of info on this is www.webmd.com), how often she takes them per day, and the cost of the medicines.

Medicare and Medicare Supplement Insurance is a difficult process to navigate for doctors' bills and hospital bills and results in a huge pile of paper for the patient. The separate file trays provide a specific place to put these documents when they arrive. A care/service provider must file with Medicare and the Medicare Supplement insurance company at the same time. Once a month or so we go through all these papers to match up the Medicare payment information with the Supplemental Insurance information to verify that everything has been handled properly. Sometimes the provider might file for Medicare, receive their payment, and then bill us for the balance. We must be able to check the Supplemental Insurance forms to see if they have been filed correctly. In most cases this was overlooked or some simple mistake was made in the submission. We then have to contact the provider's billing office, go over the charges with them, and ask them to resubmit to the Supplemental Insurance provider with the correct information. This is a hassle, but it is necessary to do. Many providers will put a hold on a past-due bill while they resubmit a claim. If not, then we have to pay them and ask them to file again. Next, we work to get them to refund what we've paid once the Supplemental Insurance pays them. Sometimes this takes months to complete. Under Medicare and Medicare Supplement rules, all payments must go directly to the provider and not to the patient. This is done specifically to take the burden of payment off the elderly. In almost all cases, Medicare and the Medicare Supplement insurance will pay 100% of the costs of doctor and hospital bills and most ancillary services. There are many things not covered by Medicare, but basic doctor and hospital care are covered. However, it is your responsibility as the primary caregiver to make sure that the paperwork is correct and that these bills are paid. The last thing you want is collection agencies calling your home looking for money because a simple error in paperwork was ignored. For you, the "care manager", Medicare is about keeping up with the paper trails.

The Prescription Drug Plans now in place for senior citizens are a maze of premiums, deductibles, co-pays, available drugs, and approved pharmacies. It is necessary to know the names, types, and quantities of prescriptions your loved one is taking. Talk to the patient's physician and discuss with him the current medications as well as any others that he expects could become necessary for the patient's care. Once you have a comprehensive list, go to www.medicare.gov and look up Prescription Drug Plans. The particular drugs offered will vary from one plan to another. Compare what prescriptions are available with each plan. Next, check prices and deductibles against the type and quantity to be taken. Medicare PDP's do not cover all medications that are taken by many Alzheimer's patients. If you find something that stands out in price, discuss generic equivalents with the doctor. We reduced Aunt Betty's monthly prescription drug expenses by an average of $950 per month. When considering Prescription Drug Plans, it is important to compare premiums, deductibles, and participating pharmacies in the area in which you live. Take your time, look the plans over carefully, and don't be afraid to ask other Alzheimer's families for their input.

As the responsible person, you should monitor ALL prescriptions being given. If your loved one goes to the hospital for an injury or illness, they will most likely be given additional medications. Sometimes these drugs may have interactions with the drugs commonly given to Alzheimer's patients. Question everything. Even though the care facility may continue giving them the medicines after they are released from the hospital, they may not always check for information regarding drug interaction. Their job is to follow the doctors' orders. A trip to the hospital might involve several doctors. One doctor may not be aware of what the other is prescribing unless the family informs him. That is why we have a 3-Ring binder for medicines. In this book we maintain a list of all drugs prescribed for Aunt Betty, how often she takes each one and the dosage amount, a printout of the drug information (including benefits, side effects, and other drug interactions), a picture of the pill, a listing of the date and doctor that prescribed it, and how long (if known) she might need this particular medicine. We use this to discuss any new medicines or changes in medication that might be warranted with any doctors who treat Aunt Betty. Mistakes involving medications do sometimes occur in even the best facilities. For this reason, we'd rather be safe than sorry.

We have covered Medicare, Medicare Supplement, and prescriptions. Since Aunt Betty lives in a memory care center, the most time-consuming part of the paperwork occurs because of these three categories. However, they also represent the lease expensive part of her care in terms of cash outlay.

In our search for the best place for Aunt Betty to reside, we had several options. I have described the conditions in several of the places we visited. Some were good and some were not. That being said, we did not find a significant difference in the cost of Alzheimer's care facilities. Ask to see a copy of the tax determination statement for any facility you visit. This is a form letter written by their corporate financial executive stating the percentage of the cost of care that is specific to medical necessity. This allows you to determine how much of the cost is deductible on taxes as medical expenses. Depending on your specific situation and the source of the money to pay for your loved one's care, this can be a significant issue to consider.

For routine out of pocket expenses we have found that a debit/credit card tied to the checking account in Aunt Betty's trust fund gives us the flexibility and documentation that we need. Our goal is to eliminate handling cash. Whenever we take Aunt Betty out of the Center for lunch, for a manicure and/or pedicure, to buy clothes, or whatever else we do for her, we pay with the debit card. Only the portion of the expenses belonging to her are included on the card. We keep all receipts. Any returns or credits are put back on the debit card and these receipts are kept, too. In this way, no cash is handled and there is no question about where any of the money was spent. If we lose a receipt, the bank still has a record of the purchase.

The final documentation we maintain is for consolidation of information. We use two methods:

(1) financial tracking software and
(2) a simple ledger worksheet.

We download all account and investment information from Aunt Betty's bank on a monthly basis. The software allows us to categorize expenses for tax and non-tax purposes and to track spending in the various categories we have established for our needs. This makes tax preparation much easier at the end of the year. We have also chosen to put some of this information in a simple ledger style notebook for reference that can be included with the trust fund documentation. This method works well for us.

Record keeping and cash flow management are two necessary factors in caring for one with Alzheimer's. Contact a qualified Attorney and Accountant to help you get set up and organized from the beginning of this journey. It is much easier to start out right and adjust as you go along, than to realize you have made some serious oversights and have to backtrack to correct them.

ALZHEIMER'S: Where Do We Go From Here?

CHAPTER 7

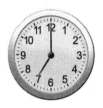

Different Emotions and Approaches

ALZHEIMER'S: Where Do We Go From Here?

CHAPTER 7

Different Emotions and Approaches

In most cases the spouse will be the primary caregiver for the one with Alzheimer's. My heart aches for some of the spouses we know who are watching helplessly as their life's partner is stolen away. Several of these couples have been married 50 years or more. Two couples have shared over 60 years together as husband and wife. Each person has to handle the disease in the way they feel is best. Last summer one woman chose to move into the home with her husband. She sold most of her possessions to move into one room with the man she loves. At that time she appeared completely fine mentally. However, as time has passed she, too, has begun having problems with short-term memory. Another delightful woman in her eighties moved her husband of 64 years into the home. She comes every day from a nearby assisted-living facility to visit her precious husband. Last week I watched a man come for his daily visit with his wife. He proudly showed off two large framed pictures. One was of him and his wife on their wedding day. The second picture was an elegant portrait of her as a young woman. His eyes beamed with pride as he announced that day was the 56th anniversary of their wedding. How it must hurt to be the spouse who does not have Alzheimer's – to be the one who goes home alone after every visit. We've also seen new couples form among the residents in the home. In situations where both people have lost their spouses, this seems sweet. For those whose spouses are still alive this only adds to the pain of the spouse without the disease. Imagine the emotions of a husband or wife as a mate walks hand in hand with another while he/she is left standing on the sidelines as the forgotten spouse of 50 or 60 years. Perhaps more heart wrenching than watching the love of your life slip away because of Alzheimer's is watching them slip away with someone else who's taken your place. Alzheimer's is an especially cruel end to a marriage. As a bystander, I find this part of the disease one of the saddest.

Our family's experiences with Alzheimer's disease have been from the perspectives of sister and niece. We are an exception to the norm among the other families whose loved ones reside in the Center. For the people whose spouses are no longer living, the responsible parties are usually their children. In a few cases, grandchildren act in this capacity. Aunt Betty is the only resident from approximately 100 people whose sister and niece oversee her care. As a result of this difference, there are times when the emotions are difficult to handle. Finding yourself in a position where you're responsible for a sick spouse, parent, or even grandparent is a more natural and foreseeable outcome than being responsible for an older sister or aunt. The relationships are so different. We never imagined that we might one day be in the position we now are as a result of Alzheimer's. The knowledge that we are the people Aunt Betty trusted to look out for her wellbeing puts enormous pressure on us to do all we can to protect her and provide for her. Having responsibility for her physical and emotional care combined with the need for wise fiscal decisions is a demanding job. To suddenly have to make these kinds of decisions for someone whose business affairs were, for the most part, previously private to us left us feeling quite uncomfortable at first. Yet, Aunt Betty chose us because she trusted us. We, therefore, want to do all we can to validate her confidence in us. Our lives have changed drastically as a result.

It's extremely difficult to put into words how we've felt at times. Aunt Betty has never been a burden. We love her and are happy to be able to help her. Though we've never viewed her as a burden, certain aspects of the situation have been burdensome. For instance, we've struggled to balance our lives so as to have ample time with Aunt Betty but not neglect the rest of our family or our other responsibilities. When there's just not enough time to fit everything in, what do we leave out? Aunt Betty has always been the number one priority. That was

fine for a while, but we can't continue that way indefinitely. As a result of this struggle, many conflicting emotions have arisen.

I have felt love, sadness, grief, and compassion. At
the same time I've felt anger, frustration, resentment,
and irritation. I know that Aunt Betty has enjoyed many
material possessions but has been starved for affection
and acceptance for much of her adult life. She always
tried to fill the void she felt with things. We all love
her and that motivates us to do as much as possible for
her. A certain satisfaction comes from being able to
fill her last days with love instead of stuff. Alzheimer's
provides a daily reminder of the importance of living in
the moment. I look at Aunt Betty and am saddened by
the realization that today may be the best day she will
ever again experience. She may awaken tomorrow and
the disease will have stolen away more of her identity
than today. Then there's always the fear of her falling.
It seems that broken bones resulting in immobility are
a common occurrence among those with Alzheimer's.
Once such an injury is sustained, the person is never
again the same. We've known several people who've
died soon after taking that kind of fall. Aunt Betty is
very unstable when she walks without her walker, and
yet she forgets to use it at least half of the time. She also
has severe osteoporosis. During the last year she has
suffered with stress fractures in her back and hip and a
broken rib. These have all happened from minor mis-

haps but her bones are so brittle that any slip or stumble has the potential for a break. We live with the constant reality that a phone call could come at any time informing us that she's fallen and broken a hip or leg. This reality compels us to continue to want to be with her as much as we can while there's still time. Another consideration is that she could awaken tomorrow or next week and suddenly have no memory of us. We routinely watch family members or long-time friends come for visits with the other residents when the resident has no idea of their names or connection to them. There might come a time when we have that same experience with Aunt Betty. That's another reason we want to make the most of each day while the opportunity still exists. When we think about what may be ahead, the emotions that are foremost in our hearts and minds are love for Aunt Betty, compassion for her condition, and sadness for all that she's already lost. Grief also fills our hearts because we know that she is really dying a slow death.

This combination of emotions would be hard enough to handle, but the story doesn't end there. On the opposite end, there are times when she becomes agitated and curses at us, accuses us of mistreating her, and tells us how unhappy she is living in the Center. My mother and I've spent hours and hours shopping for her trying to find pretty clothes or searching for things to decorate her room. Sometimes we walk in for a visit and she complains about how long it's been since she had anything new to wear or she tells us how ugly everything is in her room. If we try to remind her of some of the things we've bought for her, she insists that she's had it for five or six years. It's frustrating to think that we've tried so hard to do nice things for her but she can't remember. Some days we feel like we're beating our heads against a brick wall. After carrying her out to lunch and spending several hours in the mall shopping with her, it's not unusual for her to call later the same night and tell us she feels lonely because she's seen none of her family in over a week. When we think about all that doesn't get done in our lives like taking care of home or stopping at the grocery store because we spend so much time focusing on Aunt Betty, it's incredibly frustrating to realize she's unable to even comprehend all we do for her. There will never be a time when she understands how much we've given up for her and never a time to appreciate it. This causes me to sometimes feel resentment towards her even though I know she doesn't understand. At that point I realize we must choose to do what's right simply because we love her and we know it's the right thing, despite her not knowing.

Many days I stay three or four hours with Aunt Betty and plan to leave when she goes to dinner. I often try to explain that I need to go so I can prepare dinner for my family. She doesn't like it when we don't stay to eat with her. It's not unusual for us to hear a sarcastic little comment such as, "Well, thanks for squeezing in five or ten minutes for your aunt today. Why don't you come again when you can stay a while?" On those days I feel irritation.

Finally, there are times when anger is the most prev-alent emotion I have. One day my mother called me and all I could hear on her end of the phone were sobs. Frightened half out of my mind, I frantically asked what was wrong. She had taken Aunt Betty out to the nail salon. All was going well until Aunt Betty started insist-ing that she had to go back to our hometown to sell their mother's home. When Mom explained that had already been done, she became irate and started accusing Mom of stealing her inheritance. Aunt Betty had no recol-lection of having served as executor of Grandmother's estate years earlier. The conversation was filled with profanity and nasty names for my mother. Mom was devastated and called me to meet them. She was crushed by the cruel, and obviously untrue, things Aunt Betty said. That was just one experience, but there have been others when one or more of us have been reduced to tears by Aunt Betty's ranting. Knowing all that Mom has done for Aunt Betty and that her own health has suffered as a result of all the stress, my only reaction to episodes such as the one I described is anger. Roll all the things we've felt into one package and it's easy to understand what a roller coaster of emotions the family of an Alzheimer's victim feels.

In our family there are five of us who are closely involved with the day in and day out care of Aunt Betty in one way or another. If each of us has our own internal struggles with the emotions, multiply those feelings by five and relationships can quickly become strained. My mother is a perfectionist who gives 100 percent to everything she attempts. I am a much more relaxed person who tends to never do today anything that can wait until tomorrow. Now consider that Mom's relationship has been much different with her sister through the years than mine. For the last few years Mom talked to Aunt Betty on the telephone at least three or more times per week while my phone conversations were much less frequent. Aunt Betty still sees me as a child though I am a middle-aged woman with a grown child of my own. My days were already filled with far too many commitments outside of my home before we moved Aunt Betty to be close to us. Mom, on the other hand, did not have as tight a schedule to keep. When times have been most difficult with Aunt Betty, my reactions have sometimes been very different from my mother's. Mom has often felt that I am impatient with Aunt Betty. Perhaps that has been true on some occasions. I understand how much she has lost during the past couple of years. During those times when her thinking is most clear, she is aware of all she's lost, too. Naturally, she must feel sad and I feel sad for her. When she calls us crying because she feels sad, the first question is always, "Did you take your medicine so you wouldn't feel so sad?" We usually discover she has refused to take any medication and that has only added to her sadness. Still, Mom's typical response when that happens is for one of us to go rushing to see my aunt. Even though I love her dearly, I just can't always drop everything and hurry to her simply because she's sad. I feel sad sometimes, too. Everyone does, but people don't flock to us to fix the problem. I don't think it's fair for us to be expected to do that every time Aunt Betty feels sad either. If this means I'm impatient, then I stand as accused. However, I feel that Mom has allowed herself to become a victim at times, too. I've seen her so tired she could hardly keep going and yet, she continued to make her daily visits to the Center. I've also seen her leave in tears after spending much of the day with Aunt Betty who became verbally abusive to her before she left. Then I've watched her spend hours pouring over the bills and paperwork for Aunt Betty's care once she finally made it home.

During a counseling session our counselor told us that it was normal to feel a variety of emotions. "After all," she said, "You are losing someone you love one day at a time. Grief and anger are normal parts of the process." I thought about her statement for a few days and then came to a conclusion that really helped me understand my personal feelings. I felt that it was my mother we were losing, not Aunt Betty. Mom was so overwhelmed with all she was doing that she had little time for much else. It was killing her both physically and emotionally. I finally understood why I felt so irritated with Mom. We've spent hours discussing our feelings since then and both realize why we each react the way we do. Mom and I have always been very close and have always talked freely about everything, but this situation has presented some unique challenges. Those challenges have caused our relationship to be quite strained at times. Fortunately, we've worked through the hard times and things are fine again.

Everyone comes into a new situation with emotional baggage based on his past experiences. Reactions are largely based on those experiences in addition to the person's basic personality makeup. For example, is he more sympathetic or critical? Does he get irritated easily or is he slow to anger? Learning to accept each other's personality differences is important for an Alzheimer's family in order to prevent hurt feelings and strained relationships.

Finally, we've learned there is no one correct way to deal with Alzheimer's. Every day is a new day with its unique happenings. Sometimes it's more like every minute is a new minute because things can change so drastically within a very short time. We've watched lots of others try to deal with some of the same things we've found difficult to handle. Everybody's response is different. Sometimes people seem to react better in one situation but totally fall apart in another. Even those who have been trained to deal with the disease can have rough days, and they don't have the same emotional attachments to those who are sick with Alzheimer's as the families do. Naturally, it has to be difficult for us. Remember no one handles the obstacles correctly every time. Continue to love the person with the disease and just do your best. Having negative feelings at times doesn't make a family member a monster. It simply means you're human and you're dealing with a difficult and stressful situation. I want to be able to look back on this time with no regrets and know we did all we could do. No, we won't get it right every time; but if we lovingly give our best, what more can we do?

ALZHEIMER'S: Where Do We Go From Here?

CHAPTER 8

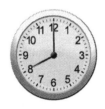

Taking Care of Yourself

CHAPTER 8

Taking Care of Yourself

"Alzheimer's is not a sprint. It's a marathon." That statement was made by a social worker during a family counseling session. It took a while for its meaning to sink in fully. She was encouraging our family to find a balance between caring for my aunt and still maintaining a life for ourselves. A sprinter focuses on speed for a short distance but soon runs out of strength. Just as a marathon runner trains for endurance, an Alzheimer's family must approach this disease with the long run in mind. As I've stated previously, we visited Aunt Betty almost every day during the first year after moving her into the memory care center. We had little interaction with friends outside the center. It often felt as if our lives were spinning out of control. There was little time for anything or anyone other than Aunt Betty. We all began to feel exhausted and totally stressed-out. We finally realized that it would be impossible to continue at the same pace. If we don't take care of ourselves, we might not be able to continue caring for Aunt Betty. We love her and hope she's around for many more years. Alzheimer's can be a long, slow process. The best way to plan for Aunt Betty's long-term care is to take care of ourselves so we'll be able to take of her.

The most important, and often most neglected, area of concern for us has been diet and exercise. Weight control has always been a struggle for our family. Unfortunately, our first response to stress is to eat. During the past 16 months, we've all gained weight. The schedule we've kept has made it difficult to plan and prepare healthy meals. Too often we've stopped at fast-food restaurants where we've grabbed high-fat, high-calorie meals. The result has been not only weight gain, but increased cholesterol levels. Unhealthy eating leaves us feeling tired and sluggish. Exercise is not an option when you feel so exhausted. That further complicates the health risks. While it's not easy, we've learned that taking time to eat a healthy diet and to exercise is essential if we're going to be able to finish the marathon called Alzheimer's disease.

Another area we've struggled with involves relaxation time. In order to adequately tend to Aunt Betty's needs, we have to allow ourselves time away from the Center. There's nothing wrong with taking time for lunch with a friend or a weekend trip to the beach. Time away should not be accompanied with guilt. Other families struggle with this same issue. It isn't negligent to miss visiting for a few days to do something for yourself. For one's own sanity and well-being, it's essential to take time for yourself.

As I've observed some of the symptoms of Alzheimer's, I've realized that learning to walk away for a few minutes is necessary at times, too. For example, Aunt Betty occasionally becomes upset about certain topics. She questions us about these topics. If we tell her the truth, she becomes angry. If we attempt to divert her attention, she gets even angrier. Sometimes she can be extremely hurtful with her reactions. There's no reason we have to stand still and take the abuse. Our walking away helps her calm down and prevents us from leaving in tears. Learning to walk away when necessary is another very important part of taking care of one's self.

We all enjoy feeling pampered. When dealing with someone with Alzheimer's, it's even more important to take time for pampering. An hour-long trip to the nail salon for a pedicure or manicure can help you feel relaxed and be money well spent if you walk out feeling good about yourself. Your focus does not always have to be the Alzheimer's patient only. Remember that you're important, too.

In the beginning, we felt like we could skip support groups since there are five of us in our family who are involved in tending to Aunt Betty's needs. In a way, we felt like we have our own support group. While it is true that we can all help each other, a support group would have been beneficial to us, especially in the beginning.

The advantage of such a group is that you can learn from the experiences of others who are further along in the journey. You can learn what to expect and get advice on how to face the challenges ahead. We've learned so many things by trial and error. If we'd been involved in a support group, we might have found the road a little less bumpy. Support groups are usually available at churches, community centers, facilities specializing in memory care, and nursing homes. Check your local yellow pages for groups in your area.

If you're not comfortable in a group setting, a private session with a licensed counselor or pastor could prove helpful. Our family met with the social worker on staff at the Center. She is a trained counselor, too. She really said very little, but knew the questions to ask to get us talking about our feelings. Once we started talking, she listened. When we were finished, she assured us that the emotions we all felt were quite normal. She made one or two suggestions about how to proceed. We left feeling much better. Sometimes all we really need is someone to listen and a counselor can do that in a more intimate setting than a support group can provide.

We have gained great insight from talking to families of other residents during our visits. It's interesting how attached we've grown to some of them. The funny thing is that in many cases we don't even know each other's last names, but we share a bond that most people don't understand. Most of my friends don't realize how much my life has changed since Aunt Betty moved here. They think she lives in a home where she's taken care of and we visit once or twice a week for an hour. How hard could that be? They don't understand how much is required of us. That's where other families facing the same struggles can be most helpful. We all speak the same language and share the same pain. We can all learn from each other and encourage one another. Encouragement from people who have walked the same path goes much further than from people who have no idea of what you're facing. If you have a loved one dealing with Alzheimer's, seek out other families who are also dealing with it. Be transparent about your experiences and you will become a tremendous support system to each other.

Finally, make it a priority to have relationships with others who have no connection with Alzheimer's. Everything in your life does not have to be about the disease. For your own good, develop friendships with people who can provide an escape. Learn to enjoy spending time with others who don't discuss the disease with you. An escape is essential for your mental, physical, and emotional health.

Sometimes loving someone else means loving yourself first. If you don't learn to make yourself and, specifically, your health, a priority you will never be able to take care of anyone else. Love yourself first and you'll be better able to love that person with Alzheimer's. Remember that he or she needs you. You can't be available to others if you constantly neglect yourself.

CHAPTER 9

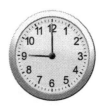

Finding Humor And
Enjoyment Wherever
Possible

CHAPTER 9

Finding Humor and Enjoyment Wherever Possible

There is so much sadness and loss for Alzheimer's patients and their families. It is important to look for fun wherever possible. Our family has been blessed to have my aunt in a place where she is given plenty of opportunities for enjoyment. Since we never acted as her caregivers at home, our perspective is probably much different than those who are providing 24-hour at-home care. It's easier for us because so many activities are planned by the activities' staff in the memory care facility.

There are parties for all the holidays. These parties usually involve special snacks and entertainment. The residents enjoy them and the families do, too. Each month there is a party for all who have birthdays that month. Families sometimes bring cakes for individual birthdays and share them with all the residents. At Thanksgiving all the families are invited to come for a big traditional turkey dinner. Each family sits together with their loved one and enjoys a wonderful meal complete with white linen tablecloths and beautiful fall centerpieces. This has been one of our favorite experiences because it was so much like the Thanksgiving and Christmas meals we've shared together before Alzheimer's took over so much of our lives. It seemed so normal. Along with parties, special outings provide enjoyment for the residents and their families. Sometimes family members are invited to go along on these outings. We've been to Senior Day which is organized and sponsored by our county for senior citizens. They experience an old-fashioned county fair with games, hot dogs, cotton candy, clowns, and balloons. We've also been to the park for picnics and to the county rodeo. At other times, Aunt Betty has gone on outings without us. She's been to a Christmas Open House, to a local restaurant for lunch, and to an area church for a special senior citizens program, to name just a few of the outings. All these parties and outings have been good times despite the disease.

With time, favorite memories fade. It is important to make as many new memories as possible. Even though the Alzheimer's sufferer will not remember them for long, the family will. No one is promised tomorrow. The Bible says our lives are like a vapor that appears for a little while and then vanishes away. Alzheimer's provides a constant awareness of this truth. It is important to learn to live in the moment. We love to see Aunt Betty have a good time. She may not remember it tomorrow or even later today, but every moment she is smiling is a good one. We will remember those times long after she will.

We take pictures of everything. My husband also video-tapes Aunt Betty with our family. Mom puts all the pictures in a beautiful scrapbook. She carries the book for Aunt Betty to see each time a few new pages are added. This has been a wonderful idea for two reasons. It will provide us with lasting memories of the happy times and it reminds Aunt Betty that she has enjoyed her time in the Center. She usually comments about how happy she looks in all the pictures. She also enjoys showing her album to her friends since they are in the pictures, too.

A few months ago my mother was suffering with hip and leg problems. It was painful for her to walk. During that time she needed to go to Wal-Mart for a few things. We decided to pick up Aunt Betty and take her with us. She has back problems and can't walk for a long time either without discomfort. So off we went with two women who were unable to walk around the store. We put Aunt Betty in the store's wheelchair and Mom rode the motorized cart. I pushed Aunt Betty. We spent almost three hours in the store that day. Aunt Betty laughed at my mother riding that cart. At one point, Mom even pushed her in the chair by pulling up behind her with the cart. My aunt thought it was hysterical that the two of them were still shopping in spite of their aches and pains. We all three laughed and had a great time. I'm not sure if Aunt Betty remembers that now, but Mom and I do. That's a new memory that we'll cherish for years to come.

We've had family gatherings at the home as well as at restaurants and our homes. Last Easter we reserved the private dining room at the Center and stopped after church services for fried chicken to go. We had a wonderful Easter lunch together as a family. When my brother came to visit from another state, we all met at my parent's home for a great time sitting together on their patio. Recently when a cousin visited from out of town, we enjoyed a meal together in one of the most popular restaurants in town. We take advantage of opportunities to gather as a family and, of course, Aunt Betty is an important part of those gatherings.

Alzheimer's hurts and sometimes it brings tears. For that reason, it's important to learn to laugh at the funny things that happen, too. Having discussed this with other families, we realize laughter is necessary to survive this experience. As parents of young children, most of us enjoyed watching our children play. Many of their words and actions are indelibly written upon our hearts as precious memories to cherish. Often those memories evoke laughter as we remember how innocent little children are. To laugh at their actions is not to make fun of them. The same is true of people with Alzheimer's since they return to a childlike state of mind. Many similarities exist, including the innocence of a child. There's a big difference between making fun of people with Alzheimer's and laughing at the cute things they sometimes say or do. Here's a great example. My aunt has always been a neat, organized person who never wanted any clutter around her. If something's left out of place, she still has to get up and put it away. Now that she uses a walker to help her get around, the walker is often one of the things she puts away. She's so cute walking down the hall to the dining room or activities room. As soon as she gets where she's going, that walker is parked neatly by the wall in an out-of-the-way spot. Then she walks over to her seat at the table or to a comfortable chair. She often forgets it when she gets up to move again and off she goes. It's funny to watch her "park" that thing, especially since she has "parking areas" in each room where she always puts it. She's always been strong and healthy and prided herself on her excellent physical condition. Even now she tells us that she only plans to use that "old thing" (a.k.a. her walker) for another week or two because she thinks it's slowing her down. That's funny. It's okay to laugh when it's funny.

I know another woman who's always loved gardening. She routinely pulls up any newly-planted bedding plants in the courtyard because she says the weeds are taking over. Her sweet daughter-in-law comes and replants them each time. We all enjoy laughing at that situation.

One of the male residents loves to take off his shoes and throw them over the fence. One day when he'd done this, he came back in with muddy socks and told me that he needed new shoes because his old ones had lost their spring. He said he no longer had any spring in his step.

At his age, that's to be expected. I laugh every time I remember that day.

On one visit to the home, my mother, daughter, and I were all sitting around a huge ottoman in the middle of three sofas. Five or six of the residents joined our circle. We decided to prop our feet up on the ottoman and discussed how good it felt to do so. It was fun to watch how much pleasure that activity provided. All of a sudden one of the women in the group started laughing as she looked at my 19-year-old daughter. She said, "Hey, you don't look old enough to be in this group." All the ladies in the group chuckled along with her. That was cute and the laughter made us all feel better.

Aunt Betty and her best friends are the more coherent residents in the home and they sometimes get irritated with some of the others. During one of my visits a woman repeatedly asked Aunt Betty, "Where are we?" At first, she answered her correctly. After being asked several times, she responded, "How many times are you going to ask me that? I just told you two minutes ago." Finally when asked, she replied with the name of another city far away. Then she looked at me, rolled her eyes, and gestured to me that the other woman was crazy. She's always been a bit sarcastic and she still is. Her reaction was hilarious. When I told my other family members about that later, we all enjoyed a good laugh. The old adage says "Laughter is the best medicine." It's okay to laugh. Sometimes that's what gets us through the day.

One of the best parts of the past year has been the new friends we've made as a result of Alzheimer's. We've met some fantastic people who are suffering with the disease. We've fallen in love with many of the residents in the home. They are such precious people who all respond to kindness. It is so rewarding to be able to stop and pat one of them on the shoulder or call out a friendly greeting as we see them. The families of so many of the other residents have also become friends. We look forward to seeing certain ones when we visit my aunt. Several of the staff have become close friends. Many conversations and laughs have been shared during our time there. Friends make any situation more pleasant.

As a Christian, I believe that the most joy in life is found in giving yourself to others. My daughter and I find such pleasure in doing little things for our friends with Alzheimer's. Sometimes we take bite-sized candy bars to one or fried jalapenos to another. My daughter, Leigh, is the most compassionate person I've ever known. She loves people of all ages, but she has a special place in her heart for older people. When we visit my aunt, Leigh goes throughout the building checking on all her friends. If someone is missing, she goes to find out what's wrong. Leigh has a friend who struggles with depression and spends much of her time in her room still dressed in her robe. My daughter can visit with her for a few minutes and encourage her to come out of her room. On one visit I overheard her tell Leigh that she was her best friend there. There are several residents who no longer talk much but they respond to her. They see her coming and their faces light up. They reach out for her and start talking. She hugs and kisses them and they look forward to her visits. It's interesting to see that they don't always respond to their own families the same as they do to Leigh. By looking for ways to give to others, we are also receiving the satisfaction of helping another person. This, too, has helped us find enjoyment in the face of Alzheimer's.

CHAPTER 10

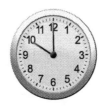

Still Alive With
Alzheimer's

CHAPTER 10

Still Alive With Alzheimer's

Can anything good be said about Alzheimer's? Surprisingly, we've learned the answer is yes. It is true that it destroys, steals, and kills, but our experiences have taught us that there are some bright spots in the midst of all the sadness. Life is a wonderful teacher. We've learned many important lessons about life from the experience of caring for Aunt Betty and observing her and her new friends.

First, I realized that there is an awareness of God that lasts long after an Alzheimer's victim is able to remember much else. While Aunt Betty was still living in the first facility and we were preparing to move her to the memory care center in our area, we had our first opportunity to interact daily with those living with the disease. We fell in love with those precious folks almost immediately. They were all so cute that we really hated to leave them behind. We enjoyed watching them greet one another throughout the day. Every time they introduced themselves and were so pleased to be meeting someone new. Each person was completely unaware that they'd met before. Due to the overmedicating she was experiencing at that time, my aunt was in the same condition. Fortunately, within two weeks in the new center her thought processes became much clearer. Despite everyone's confusion, when they'd see us walking into their residence, they'd all wave to us and several would call out "Hi there, doll" or "You know I've always loved you." We stayed with them 11 days and became acquainted with each one's sweet personality.

One day we were sitting with them at a table where they were coloring pictures. Mom started singing "Jesus Loves Me." Even the ones who had nodded off suddenly sat up straight and sang out with a new alertness. Realizing how much they enjoyed singing, Mom continued with other hymns she thought they might know. For the next 30 minutes we sang old hymns together. I watched with amazement as they remembered all the words to song after song. At times their beautiful faces would wrinkle as they strained to remember a line here or there, but the words all came back to them eventually. I was overcome with emotion as I heard them sing such songs as "The Old Rugged Cross" and "How Great Thou Art." I shared this story with a friend whose father has Alzheimer's. I told her how incredible it was to realize that even in that compromised condition they still had an awareness of God and His existence. She responded, "Wow! You know that also confirms that God has not forgotten them either. Even in the middle of Alzheimer's, they're still in His hand." The Bible says that God will never leave or forsake us. I learned from that early encounter with those dear people that God walks with a person through Alzheimer's, too.

"To love, honor, and cherish till death do you part" are such simple words committing one's self for a lifetime. When we stand in front of a minister as young, healthy people and take those vows, it is impossible to anticipate some of the heartaches that may be ahead. I've already recanted stories of some of the couples we've met who are dealing with the heartaches of Alzheimer's. Now I want to include a couple who has been one of my favorites. To protect their privacy, we'll call them Robert and Elizabeth. They moved into the Center over a year ago. Robert had been suffering with Parkinson's disease for a number of years. He was confined to a wheelchair most of the time and received all his meals through a feeding tube. Speaking was difficult for him, too. His beautiful little wife is one of the sweetest people I've ever met. Elizabeth was so proud of her husband of 61 years. She loved to tell us about his naval career that included surviving the Japanese attack on Pearl Harbor. As Robert's health declined, Elizabeth spent more and more time sitting at the foot of his bed. She came out of the room for short periods only to get a little exercise or for her meals. She'd always say, "Well, I need to go back and check on Papa Bear." Robert passed away a few months ago. Elizabeth decided to stay at the Center. We all love her dearly so we were thrilled that she stayed. Even now, she speaks often of her husband. She smiles as she talks about how good looking he was or tells the story about how they met. They shared a rare kind of love for many years. Elizabeth provides a beautiful picture for everyone who knows her of what it means to live out one's marriage vows. Even after death, it is obvious that she still loves, honors, and cherishes her "Papa Bear" as much as ever if only through her memories now.

I wish all young mothers could spend one day in a memory care facility. I've always known that a mother impacts her children's lives in ways that will continue throughout their lives. However, I had no idea of just how deep that impact goes before Aunt Betty moved into the Center. We've been fascinated by the number of people who walk around looking for their mothers. Just as a small child finds comfort in his mother's presence, many people with Alzheimer's seem to need that same comfort. I suppose the nurturing they received as young children is something they again desire as they return to a second childlike stage. As a mother, I've found this to be a good lesson on the importance of my words and actions in shaping who my daughter will be even in her old age. I wish all mothers could understand how far reaching their influence will be in the lives of their children. I suspect such knowledge would cause many to make changes that could result in much happier homes.

Aunt Betty was fortunate to have a roommate that she grew to love. Since I began writing this book, her roommate passed away. Her death was a hard blow to Aunt Betty. She has grieved deeply over the loss. Though she and her roommate sometimes argued like two sisters, they still enjoyed each other's company. If one was out of the room, the other was usually close behind looking for her. During Bev's last days, Aunt Betty stayed close to their room, checking on her often. She sat by her bed, kissing and talking to her. Bev reached out, patted her on the back, and puckered up to return her kisses long after she was able to speak any more. One of the staff commented on what great friends they had been and what a pair they were together. She said, "I hope that when I get to that point, I'll have a friend like that there for me, too. That's what girlfriends are for." Aunt Betty and Bev taught us some important lessons about friendship. From their example, we learned the importance of being real. Each of them said exactly what came to mind. There was never any pretense. We learned to forgive and forget and the importance of looking out for each other's wellbeing. They taught us the importance of laughing and crying together as each shared memories or worries. Finally, we learned the importance of "being there" until the end.

Sometimes there are detours in life that seem horrible at the time, but upon retrospection we realize they also brought blessings. I know it sounds strange to say, but Alzheimer's has been that way for Aunt Betty. I've described many of the unpleasant things about the disease. Now I want to share some of the positive things that have happened. Before the onset of the disease, Aunt Betty spent most of her days alone in her home watching her husband come and go. She was extremely unhappy. She loved her next door neighbors and saw them regularly. As her condition worsened, their attitudes toward her became more negative. She went to church every week, but that provided only two hours per week with other people. She had a family member who came to see her until my uncle began to put the puzzle pieces together regarding the money the relative was stealing from her.

Since moving into the memory care facility, Aunt Betty has nine family members living close to her. She is visited at least four days per week. She and my daughter, Leigh, are alike in many ways. They're both extremely affectionate. Aunt Betty loves to hug and kiss Leigh. It tickles her to think that my mother and I might be jealous of the two of them. She goes shopping, out to lunch, and on various outings. She enjoys a variety of activities at the Center every day. She has many good friends that she loves. She spends time visiting with her friends in their living area and dining room. She enjoys a balanced diet that she no longer has to prepare. The staff members hug and kiss her and she knows they love her. The sad truth is that Aunt Betty has a much higher quality of life now with Alzheimer's than she did before the disease.

Life is a gift from God and, therefore, something to be valued. I am sad to say that I think our modern-day culture has forgotten this fact. Too often I've heard jokes that ridicule people with Alzheimer's or portray them as a drain on society. They are presented as no longer having any worth. Nobody would ever think of ridiculing a cancer patient or someone with heart disease. Those are diseases no one would ever hope to have. The same is true of Alzheimer's. Each of these diseases chooses its own victims. The victim of Alzheimer's is entitled to the same respect as a cancer victim.

I've listened to my parents and some of their friends discussing their greatest fears about growing older. Alzheimer's is their second greatest fear while losing their mate is the greatest. They all agree that if they had to choose Alzheimer's or cancer, they'd choose cancer. In their opinions, Alzheimer's steals more of a person's dignity than any other disease.

I remember hearing a young woman refer to an older person with Alzheimer's. She said, "If I ever start to act like that, somebody put a pillow over my head." Obviously, she's never loved a person with the disease. If she had, she'd never feel that way. She'd be as offended as we were by her insensitivity in making such an unkind statement. The many wonderful people we've met who have Alzheimer's have taught me that there is always value as long as there is life. Maybe the person's conversations no longer make sense. Maybe she is unable to feed herself. She might need to wear adult diapers due to incontinence. Regardless of these changes, there is still value. I like to listen when the residents of the Center want to talk. Sometimes I can't understand, but at other times I find their stories very entertaining. I love to hear about their lives before the disease. We've met people who've spent their lives as devoted spouses and parents, doctors, lawyers, teachers, preachers, military heroes, and on and on the list goes. We've learned that they are worthy of respect for who they have been even if they're not able to be that person any longer. They're all heroes in somebody's life and as such, they still deserve to be respected.

Cognitive abilities may fade, but feelings last. That quickly becomes apparent when observing Alzheimer's victims. Since they don't really understand every situation, it's not unusual for their feelings to get hurt. Our family tries to treat all the residents in a way that makes them feel like they're somebody important. The feeling of being loved is the best feeling of all and we enjoy the opportunity to give that feeling to each of them, especially Aunt Betty. Acting like we love them is easy because we truly do love them. We miss them when we're away for more than a couple of days. They have all become our friends. They're just like all our other friends, but they just happen to have special needs.

We don't know what's ahead for Aunt Betty. We are committed to providing her with the highest quality of life possible until the end. We will continue to love her and do our best for her. Nancy Reagan gave the world an outstanding example of how to care for one with Alzheimer's while protecting his dignity. For ten years she lovingly cared for her husband, former President Ronald Reagan. As a result, she gained the admiration of people around the world. We hope that when the end comes, we'll be able to look back and know we've done all we could do and that we allowed Aunt Betty to maintain her dignity for as long as possible. I realize that my daughter is watching us and so we are setting an example for the next generation while caring for the previous one. I'm thankful that she has had the opportunity to connect with Aunt Betty and, therefore, understand more about my past, too. I hope she'll remember that we loved and helped others who couldn't help themselves. That will be part of our legacy to her. Most of all, I hope she will never lose her love for people and that she will always recognize the value of a life, especially those victimized by the dreadful disease known as Alzheimer's.